101 ROMANTIC GESTURES

Make the woman in your life feel special

Published by Glowworm Press
7 Nuffield Way
Abingdon OX14 1RL

By Connor Champion

Romantic Gestures

Transform your relationship with these thoughtful, fun, easy to use romantic gestures and watch your love blossom as you become irresistible to your woman.

This book will give you many ideas on how to show your woman how much you care for her and how much you love her with a comprehensive listing of sweet, thoughtful and simple romantic gestures which will help to spark a flame, or to keep the flame burning in your love life.

Armed with this book, you will never be stuck for ways of expressing your feelings and you will be on your way to enjoying a loving successful long term relationship with your partner.

Table of Contents

Chapter 1: How Romantic Gestures Can Help Your Love Life

We can all take one another for granted from time to time. Daily chores take over and we forget how much we love the woman in our lives, and we forget to show our love for her.

More often than not a woman wants her man to say or do the simple things, she likes to know that she is appreciated and that her man is always thinking about her and looking for ways to show his love for her.

You shouldn't have to wait for Valentine's Day to show your partner you are thinking of them. There is much more to maintaining a successful loving relationship than merely getting her a nice card on her birthday.

This book will give you many ideas on how to show your woman how much you care for her and how much you love her. It lists many sweet, thoughtful and simple romantic gestures which will help keep the flame burning in your love life.

It is true that women love to be seduced, as they get turned on in their heads first, so, choose some of the romantic gestures in this book and be prepared to enjoy the fruits of your labours.

Armed with this list of romantic gestures, your love life is bound to hit new heights. Expect to make your woman melt in your arms, fall deeper in love with you and respect you more.

Chapter 2: Simple Romantic Gestures

A woman wants to know that she is appreciated and that her man is always thinking about her and looking for ways to show his love for her. Here are some quite straightforward simple romantic gestures you can, and should, do on a regular day to day basis to show that you really care for your woman.

Open a door - it's the oldest cliché in the book - but it's one that always works - because it makes her feel special.

Put her coat on for her - it will make her feel that you are chivalrous and see her as the fairer sex.

Help your partner clean the dishes - so simple, yet so meaningful.

Clean her car on the weekend and show off your manly muscles.

Drop her off, or pick her up from work / the gym /shopping etc.

Hold hands when you're crossing a street or walking, or in the car.

Pull her seat out for her when you're in a restaurant - she will enjoy being treated like a lady.

Make her a cup of tea from time to time to show that you appreciate her.

Always remember to put the toilet seat down!

Help her with the housework - the quicker it's done, the more quality time you will get to spend together.

Help your partner prepare dinner. Help with preparing the vegetables or stirring the pots. Show some interest in what she's cooking, and how she is cooking it. After all, you will be eating it - so it makes sense to help make it the best you can.

Every day when she comes home from work give her a kiss and a cuddle and ask her how her day went.

It's the simple things that really do matter. All of these simple romantic gestures will bring you ever closer together, and lead to a more fulfilling love life for you both.

Chapter 3: Fun Romantic Gestures

These are fun things to do that don't take much effort, and each is in its own way is fun to do. You will definitely enjoy these fun romantic gestures, and so will she.

Go through revolving doors together - the tighter the squeeze the better.

Write Hello Gorgeous on the bathroom mirror in lipstick. Bet you it will still be there a week later.

Get her a stuffed animal. It doesn't really matter what type of animal it is - one thing's for sure though - she will not throw it away.

Create a special message for her using alphabet spaghetti.

Carve both of your initials into a tree, with a little heart in between e.g. CC heart GG.

Write love notes
on eggs in her
fridge.

Give her a heart shaped box of chocolates.

Candles are always a winner - any self respecting guy should regularly buy scented candles as they set the mood everywhere, from the dining room to the lounge to the bedroom. Every once in a while, light those candles and set the stage for a romantic evening.

Take her out for a picnic. The key elements for a picnic are a blanket, food and drink. You can keep it simple with plastic glasses and a cheap bottle of plonk, or you can go to town and be quite elaborate, and lay on champagne and strawberries. Either way, she'll remember the picnic fondly.

For ten minutes or so, don't let your beloved walk around the house - carry her instead. Carry her around the house no matter where she wants to go, and hopefully it will lead to the bedroom.

When you are in a karaoke bar, just before you start singing your song, tell the audience you are dedicating the song to your woman. It's a gesture she will love - and as a bonus it will also get the crowd on your side too.

Write a heart in the sand on the beach.

Bonus points if you manage to get a photo of the two of you with it.

Adopt an animal abroad in her name, and make sure what you sign up to provides sweet monthly updates on her adopted pet.

When it's your anniversary, remember what you did on your first date and re-enact it - she will love that you have remembered.

On a weekday night, get some popcorn, her favourite chocolate and cuddle up on the sofa and watch a romantic movie together that's bound to make her teary eyed. Make sure you have a box of tissues to hand, for the weepy bits.

Go on a countryside bike ride together.

Attempt to draw pictures of one another. Don't worry if you can't draw, you'll have fun and you will create a lovely keepsake.

When it has been snowing, take the opportunity to write a personal message on her windscreen e.g. CC loves GG.

Write a bucket list together of all the things that you want to do in the future with each other.

Take a class together and learn a new skill together - like cookery, painting or maybe even dance lessons.

Spend a weekend camping. Sit around your own hand made fire (she will be so impressed that you can do this) and have fun roasting marshmallows and gazing at the stars together.

All of these fun romantic gestures are easy to plan and do, and will lead to a more fulfilling love life for you both.

Chapter 4: Loving Romantic Gestures

There are many ways to demonstrate your love. Let her know you are a romantic at heart and that you really care for her by doing any of the following loving romantic gestures.

When it's a rainy day, hold the umbrella to cover her from the rain.

Go food shopping with her, she'll appreciate the company and as a bonus you get to pick your favourite foods!

Candles in the dining room will help create the right mood for a romantic dinner - it doesn't have to be for a special occasion.

Buy her a present. It could be anything - jewellery and perfume will always be welcomed but it is the spontaneity and the surprise that makes it romantic.

Make a donation
to a charity close
to her heart.

Fix your loved one her favourite breakfast in bed, and make sure there is a fresh croissant on the breakfast tray. If you can, pop a little flower in a small vase on the side of the breakfast tray for that special finishing touch.

Buy a book of love poems or go online and print one off, to read to her later - start by calling it your special poem for her.

Get her a gift certificate to her favourite store.

Surprise her by booking her a day of indulgence at a fancy spa.

Tell her to choose the soppiest chick flick she can, and go along to the movies with her. For maximum effect, don't grumble at the cinema, or on the way there or on the way back.

Read the Sunday papers in bed together.

Cook her favourite dish. Every guy should know how to prepare some basic dishes and at least one difficult one. Learn how to cook her favorite fayre and with any luck she'll treat you to dessert.

A surprise weekend getaway always works wonders.

Look into your partner's eyes and say "I love you". Say it like you mean it without trying to be funny or sounding corny.

Give her expensive handmade chocolate - personalised icing optional.

Surprise her and take her out for lunch. So few couples do this. It is the element of surprise that does the trick. It's only for an hour - at most. The rushed nature of the meeting should just heighten the sexual tensions, which could be released later.

Take her on an "official" date. After a long time together, couples tend to get lazy and skimp on the extravagant thrills of the early stages. This is something many women lament. So bring back that lost excitement and take her on a nice date. Bonus points if you take her to a fancy place where dress is formal (you know how women love dressing up).

Put a cute note
under the
windscreen wiper
on her car.

Buy her a token present. One day, for no reason, show up with a thoughtful little gift. Give her something with meaning that represents something for her. You will get bonus points if it's something she actually needs, but never told you about.

Come up with a secret sign. There's nothing that creates a world-of-two feeling more than your own private language. Create a secret gesture that means "You are adorable". Use at parties, over a family game of Monopoly, or during that dull parent teacher evening to make a connection without saying a word.

Wherever you are, whether it's walking together, in the car, or just sitting on the sofa together, make a point of holding hands. Innocent and sweet, it will remind you of that time long ago when just that was enough to get your heart racing.

Tell her she's beautiful. Women will never tire of hearing this. She will love it even more if it's unexpected. Call her randomly at work and tell her. Leave a note with this message in her purse, so that she will happen upon it some time in the day. Likewise, send her an email saying you can't wait to see her that night. She'll be so excited to see you, she might just leave work early.

Send a no reason, just because I love you text. Bonus points if you make it a little naughty.

Write her a letter. In these days of email, instant messaging and phone texting, the noble art of writing love letters has all but disappeared. This makes the act of writing a love letter even more special. So, simply write your loved one a hand written letter, making sure you date it and post it with a first class stamp, with a few kisses on the back of the envelope. Stuck for words? Not to worry - just keep it simple - a short letter saying I Truly Love You will still hit the spot - and will be kept for ever.

Dance with her. To really make it special, dance with her outdoors, in a public park. She'll feel like she's in a movie.

If there is ice on her car, take a couple of minutes to de-ice her windscreen.

Tell her you love her in a different language. Use Google translate - and choose an obscure language - so if you want to tell her you love her in Polish it is Kocham Cię or Mongolian it is Bi chamd khairtai. If those are a bit difficult and hard to get your tongue around, go for the nice and easy French words Je T'aime.

Plant a tree
together and
watch it blossom
like your love.

Plan a romantic weekend away to somewhere you
know she would love.

Go for a romantic dinner to her favourite restaurant.

When you know your partner will be having a shower,
nip into the room beforehand and steam up the
mirror and write 'I love you' on it. Let the room cool
down. The room will steam up again when she is
having a shower and when she exits the shower, she
will have a lovely romantic message waiting which is
guaranteed to make her go weak at the knees.

If you are going away on a trip and have to leave your
loved one, spray your aftershave on an item of
clothing that she can take to bed with her so that she
can feel close to you.

Leave a voicemail telling her how much you love her.

Spend a few hours collecting romantic love songs,
burn them on to a CD or memory stick and slip it into
her purse or handbag.

Place a Love Heart with the message You're Mine on her pillow at night..

If your partner listens to a radio show regularly, email the station presenter and ask them to dedicate a song to her.

On your first Christmas together make a personalised ornament for you both to hang on the tree. Then do the same every year.

Buy a packet of Love Heart sweets and find the one that says forever yours, take a picture and email it to her at work! It will make her smile that's for sure.

Get her a wristwatch and have it inscribed with a cute message such as "Our love is timeless" or "I always have time for you."

Get a pack of post it notes and on every single page write I Love You (dotting your I's with hearts optional). Now leave each post it note everywhere at her place.

Write little love notes (could be about anything) to your partner and slip them into her handbag.

Write a love note and insert it into a balloon - blow up the balloon, and write on a tag on the balloon Pop Me, and then give her the balloon

These loving gestures will lead to a more fulfilling love life for you both.

Chapter 5: Big Her Up

There are many ways to show that you truly appreciate your lady.

Praise her in public. When you are out on a social gathering with friends and family, praise your partner, describing specifically her strengths and qualities and how great you think she is.

Phone your partner out of the blue and give her a very short sweet message like "I'm glad I met you" and then that's it - don't get drawn into day to day conversation - just hang up.

Demonstrate you think about her when she's not around. Email her links to stories that you knows will interest her; especially when they're about topics that *don't* interest you.

Being sincerely interested in your significant other is essential to making a relationship last. Make it clear that you're interested in what she does, what her opinions are, and where her passions lie.

Massage her nice
and slowly –
ideally with
scented massage
oils.

Invite her to meet your folks. Our parents bring out the best and worst in us; your wanting her to experience that dynamic shows real trust and vulnerability.

Take her back to a special place you went when you started dating.

When she cuddles up on the sofa, wrap her up, especially her feet, in a soft blanket.

These supportive gestures will make her respect and appreciate you more.

Chapter 6: Say It With Flowers

Flowers are a classic way of saying I Love You, and flowers have the benefit of lasting too, serving as a constant reminder of your love for her.

Don't wait for Valentine's Day or her birthday. Be spontaneous and buy her some flowers. Make sure to be original though and pick one that she is not used to receiving, like an orchid.

Sprinkle rose petals in the bath.

Buy her a plant. Choose something like a lily, bromeliad, anthurium or gardenia depending upon the season. Whatever you do, don't buy her a cactus.

Leave rose petals as a trail, from the front door to the bedroom.

Cover the bed in rose petals.

Simple, yet timeless, flowers are always a welcome romantic gift.

Chapter 7: Thoughtful Gestures

Sometimes it isn't about what you say, it's about what you do. Yes, it is true that actions speak louder than words, and the following actions will certainly speak volumes about how much you care for your loved one.

Choose your softest most luxurious body towel and pop it into the tumble dryer the moment your partner pops into the shower. As your beloved exits the shower, be on hand to pass her the freshly warmed up towel. Don't have a tumble dryer? Simply put the towel on a warm radiator instead.

Give your partner a gentle foot massage when both of you are relaxing on the sofa. Work the whole foot and rub gently while humming your lover's favourite tune. Be gentle and don't get distracted.

Plump up the pillows so next time they will be at their maximum comfort.

At a public event where there is a PA system whether it be at a train station or a theatre or a sports event, ask the staff to dedicate a loving sentence to her.

Change the
wallpaper on your
phone to a
picture of her.

Find a quiet place in the countryside where you can
watch the sunset together.

If your partner falls asleep on the sofa cover them
with a blanket to keep them warm and secure.

Show how much you pay attention to your beloved
and surprise her with tickets to see her favourite
comedian or band.

*These thoughtful gestures will make her realise you
really care about her.*

Chapter 8: Sexy Romantic Gestures

There are many sexy things you can do that don't take much effort, and each will get your partner in the mood.

Choose your partner's favourite dessert and insist that you do the spoon feeding, teasing her as you playfully twist the spoon into her mouth.

Prepare a meal using as many aphrodisiacs you can think of. Start the meal with oysters.

Organise a sexy scavenger hunt. When your beloved comes home, have a little adventure prepared for her. Be sure to make the scavenger hunt sexual by telling her to slowly prepare herself for a night of passion. For instance, when she is in the kitchen, tell her to have a glass of wine; in the bathroom tell her to moisturise herself, then to her bedroom, put on some sexy lingerie - you get the idea.

Set the alarm for fifteen minutes earlier than usual and use that time for a morning quickie or just to cuddle. Fifteen minutes isn't going to make a difference in how rested you are, but it will make you happier all day.

Wear nothing but an apron while you cook her dinner.

Tie a ribbon around your waist or any other strategic location and be her gift for the night.

Fancy dress hire shops are not just for parties. Surprise your love one by dressing up as a policeman, cowboy, fireman etc. Act out her fantasy - or yours!

Run a bath for her. If your loved one doesn't like bubbles in the bath, then don't put bubble bath lotion in. However, if she does, then go to town, and put in five times more bubble bath lotion than normal and surround the bath with sweet smelling incense sticks. Make her feel like a Hollywood starlet. Ask her if she wants you to join her, or if she wants to relax on her own.

The final romantic gesture in the book is one that you will both remember all your lives – Give her a sensual massage. All over.

All of these sexy yet romantic gestures will work wonders for you, and lead to a more fulfilling sex life for you both.

In Summary

Romantic gestures are as old as romance itself, and there really isn't an excuse for resting on your laurels and putting in the bare minimum of effort. Your woman expects you to be inspired enough to pull out a few tricks even after you've been together for a while. Don't worry, she isn't necessarily looking for sonnets or grand gestures of a cinematic calibre.

There are plenty of romantic ideas here in this book for you. It would be incredible if you could manage to do a few of these, but more importantly it would be incredible for your partner to be on the receiving end of some of these romantic gestures.

It is important that you do find time to listen to any worries on her mind and put her at ease letting her know that you will always be there for her.

Making her feel good isn't about spending loads of money or putting hours into planning something flashy. Love is less about having sex every week. Love is less about expensive gifts. It's about being struck with the sudden desire to make her feel special in a romantic way that you know would resonate with her that she'll remember most fondly.

Finally, remember to show love for your partner at all times, so make a point of saying those three magic words to your loved one every day. Tell her how much you love her at every opportunity to make her feel special.

About the author

Connor Champion is a nom de plume for award winning author Carl Christensen; who once started and ran Slow Dating which was for a number of years the UK's favourite speed dating company. He hosted and oversaw many evenings and saw numerous relationships develop as a result of people meeting at speed dating events. During his time at the helm, he spent a lot of time asking attendees what they though being romantic means - hence this book.

Carl has since gone on to write many successful best-selling books.

I hope you enjoyed this book, and if you did, please leave a review on Amazon. Thanks in advance.